Sally
Face like a flower

BILL ANDERSON

Dent Dale Publishing

First published in July 2004 by
Dent Dale Publishing
Ebor Cottage, Whitbygate, Thornton-le-Dale,
Pickering, N. Yorks, YO18 9RY
Reprinted October 2004

ISBN 0 9547772 0 4

Produced by Freelance Publishing Services, Brinscall, Lancs
www.freelancepublishingservices.co.uk
Printed in Great Britain by Biddles Ltd, King's Lynn, Norfolk

Contents

Foreword

Sally Johnson (1974–2000)

We, those of us active in the field of learning disability, rather tend to focus on what we have done – or would like to do for people with learning disabilities.

Sally Johnson stands all that on its head. With Sally, you have to focus on what she achieved in her very short life. Indeed, what she has done for the rest of us.

This is not so remarkable because of her learning disability. Her health problems, involving a lot of pain, could have given her every reason just to stay alive or mourn the things she could have done.

Instead Sally focused, with a single-minded determination, on using her talents as an artist to raise funds for other people.

I don't know whether the words "altruism" and "empathy" featured in her vocabulary. They certainly featured prominently in her life; and the lives of those who spent time with her – and those who benefited from her fundraising were all greatly enriched because of this.

I am not surprised that as a Yorkshire lad (I was a "lad" a long time ago!) that she was a Yorkshire lass.

It was a great pleasure to be able to present her with the Gateway Gold Award – in recognition of achievements on top of her fight for survival. Her painting would have been achievement enough for most people.

This book is also a tribute to her family and friends for the support they gave and the relationship they enjoyed with a remarkable young woman.

The Lord Rix Kt, CBE, DL
President, Mencap Society

This book is dedicated to everyone who encouraged Sally to achieve her potential and live a full and happy life.

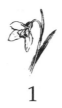

1

Overwhelming love

"Hello, little one," Sheila whispered softly. "Hello Sally."

She had often imagined this moment, and as she lay back on the pillows, her body spent from the effort of birth, she was anxious to caress the fragile bundle. After years of doubts and fears Sheila Johnson had never lost hope that she would have a child one day, Sally ... her baby. She felt it was the happiest moment in her life.

She held out her arms as the nurse placed her baby in a cot at the bottom of the bed and moved away without comment. The nurse's face was a mask, but her eyes betrayed something ... a kind of sadness.

Sheila gazed down at the baby. Such a delicate thing. A face like a flower, she thought. Sally, the child she had yearned and prayed for.

"Have you noticed anything different about her?" It was a man's voice, cold and slightly strained.

She looked up at the doctor, his dark features set in a serious expression and his manner as crisp as the white coat he wore. Sheila's eyes were drawn immediately and anxiously back to her baby. "Not really," she said. "No ... why?"

"We think she's a Mongol," he said more softly.

For several moments his words hung in the air between them. Suddenly all the ecstasy and joy began to drain away as Sheila's mind started to spin with confused thoughts. How could it be? After all the heartache of three miscarriages! She had been so careful. What had gone wrong?

She fixed her eyes on the tiny face peering from the crisp

folds of hospital linen as it seemed to turn slowly from post-natal purple to a warm suffused pink. Her Sally looked so peaceful, so beautiful … so alive.

What had happened to the baby she had carried those long, sweet, anxious months? The child she always pictured so clearly. A girl, growing up to be a real tomboy with curls or pigtails, a face kissed with summertime freckles? Now a few cold words had taken away all the joy and a glorious vision. In its place was a sad memory of a care home Sheila visited as a student teacher in the 1950s. Tears welled in her eyes as she remembered … the row of men with Down's Syndrome, slumped in chairs, left to dribble and fumble, wasting their days away in solitude and clinical indifference.

In later years, Sheila would often look back on that bleak day in the maternity ward and wonder. How different it might have been had she known then that Sally, her helpless infant, would one day become a powerful force for change? Might the ache of grief have eased? Would she have shed fewer tears for knowing that the less than perfect product of her love would touch so many lives with her talent, courage and faith?

The doctor slipped away unnoticed as the nurse returned to draw the curtains around Sheila's bed in a sham of concern for her feelings. Both had fulfilled their obligations and were glad to retreat, leaving Sheila alone with her thoughts. Those curtains felt like a barrier between her and the other happy new mothers with their "perfect" children.

Sheila wiped away her tears and reached down to gather up her child. Her baby … Sally. "It's not your fault," she whispered. "Not your fault, darling."

Despite all her sadness there was no denying an overwhelming deluge of love she felt at that moment. That indescribable force only new mothers know. Nothing had changed that. Sally was part of her, the baby she longed for. A child with a face like a flower. "Hello, little one," Sheila murmured again and again. "Hello."

Ten long, anxious days of waiting followed before she

knew for certain. A chromosome test confirmed Sally had Down's Syndrome. The first and most obvious symptom was she couldn't suckle. Each feed was a drop-by-drop struggle all day and endless nights on the busy hospital ward. New mothers came and went, too embarrassed and grateful for their own good fortune to share baby talk with Sheila. So, as the days passed, her world shrank. People she felt sure would visit stayed away. Those who came were uncomfortable and left as quickly as decency permitted. Most preferred to send cards rather than visit. Sheila pictured them agonising in shops over pictures of apple-cheeked cherubs they dare not choose. Those that arrived bore a mixture of storks and washing lines full of baby clothes and pink nappy pins. The cryptic messages inside some cards spoke volumes. "So sorry to hear ...", some wrote. "So sorry ..."

Sheila's faith, always strong, was now helping to evaporate any self-pity. It had been a shock, of course, but this was the child God had given her who needed more loving care than the other helpless newborns around her.

Sally needed her now and they would need each other for the rest of their lives. It was an enormous challenge, but Sheila knew her family and closest friends would rally around to help her face an uncertain future.

Her husband, Ken, was supportive from the start in his quiet, reassuring way. He was 58, almost 20 years older than Sheila and more the age of a grandfather than a new parent.

Ken was a widower when he and Sheila met over their mutual interest in painting, and fell in love.

"She's ours and she'll be OK," he said. "We'll do the best we can for her. She will need all the love we can give – and she'll have it."

With that promise sealed, Sheila and Ken took their 11-day-old baby home from hospital to embark on the great challenge life had given them.

Sadly others, like their elderly local doctor, had other ideas on what they should do now.

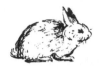

2

Warmth and understanding

"You won't want to keep her," said their elderly GP. "She'll grow up to be the village idiot. You'll walk down the street and she'll be dribbling and drooling. You'll be ashamed of her."

Poor Ken. He was a successful, contented artist in the pretty North Yorkshire village of Thornton-le-Dale. He loved his work, his wife and the countryside he had painted for 40 years. Now he had to cope with fatherhood, Sally's disability, an exhausted wife, and long nights of worry when Sally couldn't feed and wouldn't sleep. He had to fight and conquer the stressful thought that their upside-down lives would never be righted. Now their doctor was painting a grim picture, a nightmare future. Ken knew that despite his brusque manner and cruel words the doctor firmly believed his advice was in the best interests of the family.

"I'll talk to Sheila," Ken told him, knowing full well what she would say.

It was easier to say than defending a decision they had already taken and had no intention of changing.

However, they soon became accustomed to defending Sally. One elderly neighbour said it would be wiser to send her away because she could lower property prices in the neighbourhood. Another took 18 months to bring herself to look at the child, but Sheila refused to hide her. After all those years of peering into prams, envying other women's babies, she now had a pram of her own and she wanted the whole world to see Sally and love her. She was a woman with a mission, aware of the whispering she didn't want to hear. It was the long walks in the surrounding countryside, which she enjoyed so much, that helped her forget any unkind attitudes and thoughts about her baby, real or imagined. And pity was the last thing she wanted. Her hunger was for warmth, understanding and a loving acceptance of her baby.

In different circumstances village folk are always eager for a glimpse of a new baby. As it was, many avoided them but always as politely as they could. Some suddenly disappeared indoors when they saw them approaching, others crossed the road or feigned distraction.

"Well, what can you say?" they seemed to ask one another, shaking their heads in self-conscious doubt. It was 1974, a supposedly enlightened era, but for Sheila and Sally it might have been Victorian times. To many of the older generation, physical and mental disabilities were still signs of a divine retribution to be hidden, not publicly paraded. Sheila could only imagine what they might be saying: "Has she no shame, this woman? Besides, she's 40. What kind of age is that to be starting a family? Asking for trouble, that is." Sheila's imagination wasn't playing tricks. Soon the gossip was in full flow. Rumours circulated the village about terrible noises coming from their cottage. Sheila and Ken might have laughed it off as superstitious nonsense. But it was too painfully real.

"What on earth do they think I've given birth to?" Sheila demanded, through tears of frustration and a rare moment of anger.

Ken's only and immediate answer was a long, loving hug. "It will all pass over," he said. "You'll see ... don't let it get to you."

Sheila had been a primary school teacher in some of the most deprived areas of Britain before Sally was born. She had close, understanding friends, but most lived too far away for easy contact. Messages of encouragement were welcome, but no substitute for a supportive hug, an invitation for coffee, or help with the ironing. She urgently needed new friends, but where could she start? Baby groups, playgrounds? That obvious route for new mothers appeared closed to her. Sally was far too weak to attend a baby group. Besides, Sheila began to avoid being confronted by happy mothers proudly displaying their offspring. Worn down by her isolation, she found it difficult to meet anyone's gaze. She would scurry through the village, head down, seeking the safety of the front door, not feeling secure until it was closed against sympathetic stares. Yet she also was aware the real problem was a lack of understanding of Down's Syndrome.

At times she felt utterly dispirited. Yet at the bottom of that spiral of despair, prayer was the immediate answer. There was a solution. She had to be brave, trust her natural maternal instincts and be strong for Sally and their future happiness in a village she and Ken loved.

So no more self-pity or tears, she decided. No more negative thoughts about folk or herself or Sally. She decided to blank them all out – for good.

"With God's help we'll be all right," she told Sally as she pushed the pram more slowly everywhere, shoulders squared, head held high.

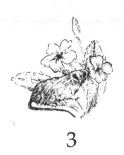

3

Village idiot indeed!

Sally became more endearing with every passing day. To those new mothers who are led to believe all happy babies sleep the day away, she would seem a rare gift. Like most with Down's Syndrome, she was so placid she could almost be happily ignored. However Sheila had spent years teaching problem children and the very idea of allowing Sally to doze away in a haze of indifference was not an option.

"You must be stimulated," she urged in conversations with a sleeping Sally. "We've got to get you interested in everything, seeing and doing things, or we might as well give up now – and we won't do that."

Ken agreed, but felt there was probably no great rush. Sally was, after all, only ten weeks old.

Undeterred, Sheila decided Sally must be coaxed to stop lying flat on her back in the pram snoozing away on their walks. She placed more pillows around Sally, propping her up so she could see what was going on around her. At first Sally was having none of it. Despite Sheila's best endeavours, she would somehow manage to slide down for a nap. Then, suddenly, when she was nearly one year old, and Sheila had almost given up hope, Sally sat up in the pram on her own and stayed up. Excited, Sheila ran all the way back to the village, tears of joy streaming down her cheeks as she burst into Ken's little studio.

"Look! Look at her!" she said, dancing round the room with Sally in her arms, while a bemused Ken looked on.

"Village idiot indeed!" she said, defiantly.

That day proved the turning point, not just a significant stride forward for Sally. It was the start of her acceptance in the community. If folk didn't look at her she could attract their attention and, hopefully, a response. Sally was never backward in coming forward and from that moment she put herself on show. Who could fail to respond to that face like a flower?

Sally soon ignited the natural warmth in the village and all the prejudices started to melt away and eventually disappear.

"Three people spoke to me today. They even said 'hello' to Sally," Sheila told Ken in the first of daily reports of every social encounter.

Of all the battles Sheila, Ken and Sally were destined to face, this was the first and the sweetest victory.

Sadly, as their love for her became stronger, Sally grew physically weaker. It also became harder to accept they might lose her. It was impossible to imagine life without her, but in moments of frightening realism it was difficult to see how she could survive. Sally had weighed a healthy 7lbs at birth, but her feeding problems soon took their toll. She swallowed only tiny amounts of milk before the effort of sucking completely exhausted her. Day and night for two years she had to be fed every two hours. Frequently, she would take only half-an-ounce of fluid then immediately regurgitate it. Sheila knew that unless Sally began to feed normally there was little chance of her survival. She borrowed medical books to see if she could learn to improve her care for Sally, but soon found that all the available literature on Down's Syndrome and its problems was depressing. It offered no real solutions. It was enough, the books implied, just to let them feed and sleep. If they failed to make it, well… maybe it was just nature's way of removing a burden. At times, as Sheila became more anxious, some people even seemed to imply it was best not to try too hard to keep Sally alive.

The situation became desperate and Sally was admitted

to hospital, where a paediatrician – the first they had seen – told Sheila and Ken: "She has such elegant eyes." But then, rather unkindly after the compliment, he added: "She'll probably grow up to be a reasonable cabbage." His best but impractical advice to Sheila and Ken was that they should have another child.

"How can some people be so insensitive? Can't they see we love her and have feelings too?" said Ken, as he comforted Sheila.

Fortunately, some health professionals could see this clearly. A new family doctor arrived in the village full of interest in Sally, always supportive and reassuring and with great warmth for the Johnsons. The only problem was that Sally objected loudly to his cold hands during examinations. The health visitor, too, was understanding and became a family friend. She quickly understood why Sheila found visits to the baby clinic so depressing.

"I can't face the comparisons," said Sheila. 'My baby weighs this. My baby can do this and that.' Not when Sally is not gaining weight."

The kindly health visitor soon elected to become a regular visitor to Sheila's house, always welcome, even if her scales were not.

After yet another disappointing weigh-in Sheila decided: "I don't need those scales to tell me how frail she is. I know she isn't putting on weight, I'm doing my best… all I can."

From then on, with Sally still struggling to feed and survive, the health visitor decided to leave her scales in the car. Somehow it paid off. Sally reached her first birthday having put on 4lbs in weight. She was only 11lbs, but she had a family who adored her; had learned to sit up; and was beginning to win lots of friendly interest from village folk – who were now aware of her battle to survive.

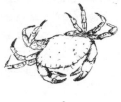

4

Chatterbox!

The next three years were among the happiest for Sheila and Ken. Sally was taken for so many walks the rubber pram wheels needed replacing twice. They were no longer the depressing excursions of the early days. People who had been aloof or indifferent seemed to delight in Sally's progress. They stopped to chat with Sheila and baby-talk to Sally, who always responded with a smile.

Sheila's immediate family were supportive from the beginning. During the critical first year when Sally was struggling to survive, Sheila's mother, Noreen, sold her home in Bridlington to move to Thornton-le-Dale. She rented a cottage nearby to be on hand and gave whatever help she could. She and Sally quickly became best friends. "Gran" always found the energy to push the pram for miles, and the imagination to keep Sally happy and interested, giving Sheila respite and time for all her other chores.

Sally also found a loving friend in Sheila's sister, Pat Spence, who was born with spina bifida and then confined to a wheelchair after suffering serious injuries in a road accident. She never complained or let life get her down, and it was from her Auntie Pat that Sally learned to make light of her own increasing health problems.

For Sheila, her loving family was an inspiration in those early difficult days of motherhood. She was able to spend more quality time with Sally, talking to her constantly, repeating words and sounds as they strolled and played together. It was no surprise that Sally spoke her first words at

11 months old: "dad, dad, dad" and "dog, dog, dog." "Gran" was just a growl and "mum, mum, mum" came much later.

Once she discovered talking was fun Sally never stopped, encouraged by everyone. She also acquired a love of picture books and music. Sheila would play a tape and put Sally in a baby bouncer so that she could "dance" to her favourite songs – wonderful for learning new words and nursery rhymes as she strengthened her leg muscles. Sally's early appreciation of her baby-bouncing music was to prove an additional strength later.

Soon Sally demonstrated a toddler's thirst for adventure even though she still couldn't walk. At 18 months she was swimming, only to give her mother a fright by doggy-paddling into the deep end at the pool in nearby Pickering.

Sally even took up horse-riding, and Saturday mornings were never quite the same again. Sheila, despite a fear of horses, bravely led Sally's hired-by-the-hour pony, Topper. It soon became a battle of wills because Topper, like Sally, had a mind of his own.

These were the idyllic summers of Sally's early childhood. Friends rented a beach chalet in Scarborough for eight weeks each year as a gift for her. She spent sun-drenched hours playing at the water's edge with special friends Eleanor Parker and Laura Coffey and others they met on the beach. They built magnificent sandcastles, rode on the donkeys, fished in the rock pools and threw bread to the seagulls.

It was a gloriously happy time for Sheila, too, as she saw her daughter being freely accepted as just another little girl at play, making friends naturally and easily. She doubted whether the other children noticed she was different. It made Sheila even more determined that Sally should live as normal a life as her health would permit.

Now every night when Ken walked through the door Sally had something new and exciting to tell him in a breathless torrent of words.

"The horse had its foal, Daddy … and we fed the ducks … and we had chocolate and Mummy said I shouldn't tell …"

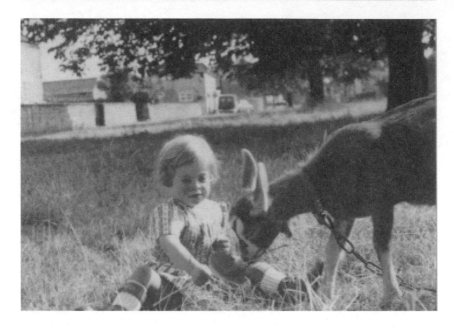

Making friends

Funny, loving, inquisitive. Who could have asked for a better daughter? But having a bright and intelligent child was one thing, making others believe and accept this was quite another. Sally attended a playgroup in Scarborough for children with disabilities. But after her third birthday, Sheila felt it was time for her to move on. She wanted Sally to mix with children from her own village, hopefully those she would go to school with later on.

She soon realised she had another struggle on her hands because Sally still couldn't walk. She shuffled about on her bottom or tummy and was still in nappies.

"I'm sorry, children have to be toilet-trained before they can be accepted," the play leader said.

Sheila persisted and the lady finally conceded, on condition Sheila accompanied Sally to all sessions. It was a difficult compromise. Sheila's aim had been to encourage Sally's independence. However there was consolation, like witnessing the delightful moment when Sally demonstrated to everyone that she was not the timid, helpless child they thought.

"Would you like me to say a nursery rhyme?" Sally asked and without waiting for an answer she launched into Humpty Dumpty ... then Jack and Jill ... and Mary, Mary ...

All the other children were amazed; the play leader impressed and delighted.

Sally flourished at the play group.

By three-and-a-half she was reading Janet and John books, and she went on to complete the whole reading scheme at home before she was old enough for the village school. Far more important, she had learnt how to get on with and enjoy being with other children; and for them to accept her. Sally's natural charm and cheerful enthusiasm was to help her to make new friends easily – throughout her life.

5

Short time to live

Sally was reading, talking and playing. She was a happy child, and full of fun, but serious doubts lingered about her health. She was making incredible progress mentally, but physically she was failing. She still couldn't walk, and her boundless enthusiasm couldn't hide the alarming fact the slightest physical effort left her exhausted. Sheila had to take her to hospital for endless tests. One day the specialist detected a worrying heart murmur; later it was gone.

"It's nothing serious," he said reassuringly. "Lots of babies are born with a heart murmur. She'll be fine." She wasn't. Her health was like a yo-yo – up and down, but now mostly down.

"I'm really worried about her," Sheila told Sally's new paediatrician. "Something isn't right."

He referred Sally to a heart specialist in Leeds for more tests. The result was devastating, so grim he could hardly bring himself to tell Sheila.

"She has only a short time to live," he said. "I'm so sorry."

Sheila was stunned and could only watch his lips as he pronounced the tragic new scenario for the family. Then something amazing happened. Sheila had seen Sally treated in the most callous way by a few health professionals. She watched as the consultant scooped Sally into his arms and held her close.

"Oh, Sally," he said, his voice choking. It was the first time anyone outside the family had shown such genuine emotion for her.

"Thank you," Sheila wanted to say. But although her lips moved, her voice failed when she desperately tried to respond to his kindness. She walked away from the hospital clutching Sally tightly to her, feeling her warmth, keeping her safe.

Sally had hypertension. There was a hole through each section of her heart, and the pressure of blood was causing irreversible damage to the blood vessels in her lungs.

Sheila couldn't look or talk to anyone. She didn't even remember driving home. She went through her household chores automatically, with a single thought running repeatedly through her head: If Sally had only weeks, days or months she must never know. There would be no time for sadness, only happy days, every day. That night, as Sally slept, Sheila sat beside the bed gazing at her tranquil face – that face like a flower – until she herself slipped into an exhausted sleep to briefly escape the heartache she hid so well from everyone.

* * * * *

Sheila and Ken knew each time Sally went to playgroup or a party, or even on the swings she so enjoyed in the park, there was a chance an accidental tumble could be fatal. Those joyful moments of freedom she loved so much were now to be bought at the price of their peace of mind. They talked about it endlessly. Should they keep Sally at home? Savour every moment? To prolong her life? Or should they let her stay the little girl they so wanted her to be?

"We should let her live her life. We can't keep her wrapped up in cotton wool," said Sheila. "She would go mad; so would we."

"I know," said Ken. "But what if something happened? We'd never forgive ourselves."

"No." She shook her head. "We'll never forgive ourselves if we don't give her a chance to live as normal a life as possible."

In the end, there had to be a sensible compromise. Swimming and riding, those two shining beacons of fun in Sally's routine, were no longer permitted. Her socialising, joining in the rough and tumble of ordinary childhood play, remained – at the cost of her parents' constant anxiety. Then, one night, as Sheila was putting Sally to bed she noticed a lump on her stomach.

"It's probably nothing," Ken reassured her. "It'll sort itself out."

"Yes. You're probably right."

But the lump remained, meaning another hospital appointment, another specialist, and more bad news. Sally required an urgent operation but that was out of the question. Her heart was simply too weak. For Sheila, whose faith had seen her through every crisis so far, the only option was prayer. She decided there was no point in a single prayer when scores could be despatched with the help of the local churchgoers. So the villagers of Thornton-le-Dale prayed as they had never done before.

Word spread and soon hundreds more were praying for the face like a flower.

The next day, the lump on Sally's stomach had disappeared. It never came back.

Who could resist such a heavenward salvo of supplication?

6

Tightrope to independence

The months passed. Sally happily celebrated her fourth birthday despite medical opinion that it could well be her last. Each calendar event was now another marker for her survival: the falling Autumn leaves, birthdays, Bonfire Night, Christmas, spring flowers and the cuddly lambs in the field opposite the Johnson cottage. The days came and went, and Sally, oblivious to her parents' concern, seemed to enjoy every minute. As Sally sat beside her mother in the tiny village Methodist Church on that crisp and sunny Christmas Day morning, singing Oh Little Town of Bethlehem with all her might, Sheila couldn't imagine a Christmas without her.

At times, Sally's infectious optimism dispelled Sheila's fears. The child's irrepressible love of life made it difficult for anyone to remain depressed in her presence. So, as they turned the pages of the calendar, Sheila and Ken tried to relax and consider the immediate future. The most pressing problem was Sally's inability to walk. Her feet and ankle muscles were weak and her pram had been replaced with a wheelchair. Her orthopaedic surgeon suggested surgical boots and knee-length callipers to strengthen her ankles. When they arrived, they were as cumbersome and ugly as Sheila had feared. She watched anxiously as Sally's tiny feet slipped so easily into the heavy boots and her legs were strapped into the steel callipers.

"They feel a bit strange!" was the only comment from Sally.

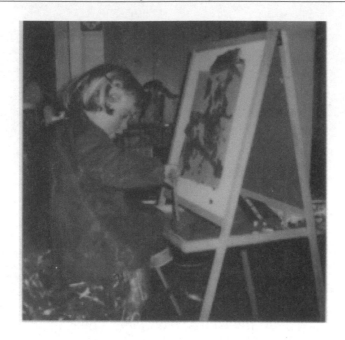

Early promise

Within months, Sally was walking … well, running, if a little clumsily. The toddler who had never been able to toddle now had a great deal of lost time and mischief-making to catch up on. It was also almost time to go to school, that momentous transition in the life of every child and parent. Sheila toured local special schools for children with learning difficulties but quickly realised they were unsuitable. Sally had so many and varied special needs, but there was little wrong with her intellect. There were also doubts of her ability to cope and progress in a school filled with boisterous children with their own special needs. They might not understand Sally's frailty during play.

Sheila decided the best solution would be a place in a mainstream school. Sally made this possible by sailing through all the IQ tests at speed. The final but crucial test at the hospital seemed to drag on for an impatient Sally. She was unable to contain herself any longer. She leapt to her feet, trotted over to a long mirror in the corner of the room and launched into her very own, delightfully expressive rendition of the Hokey Cokey. The stunned and highly amused assessor quickly conceded the village school could take such a bright and lively youngster.

At that time it was rare for children with clear special needs to be accepted into a mainstream school, but Sally's headteacher was a man ahead of his time.

"She's a first-class citizen and should be treated as such," he told Sheila. "She'll be OK. We'll look after her."

Yet no amount of reassurance could ease Sheila's misgivings as she waved goodbye to Sally at the school gate for the first time.

It was the longest morning of Sheila's life until she collected Sally at lunchtime. Her daughter's enormous smile gave her all the reassurance she needed.

"It's great, Mum!" she said. "Can I go again tomorrow?"

And so it was that Sally took her first tentative steps along the tightrope to independence.

7

A step too hard and high

Not once in her time at the village school was Sally ever mocked. Her callipers and new glasses with thick lenses set her apart. Classmates quickly accepted her. There was no bullying, no name-calling, or leaving her out of their games. Sally became what her parents had always hoped; another child in a playground full of children, making friends, learning to live life happily.

"I never thought those callipers would be such a god-send," Sheila told Ken. "The children see them and they know there's something wrong. So they give her a wide berth when they're chasing around. And when they see she needs help, they give it. They are all so caring with her."

If there was one downside to school for Sally it was maths. She was advanced in her reading, but figures remained a baffling mystery. It became a test too far, a challenge she could not win, no matter how she tried.

These were pioneering times for special needs children in mainstream schools with so much to learn on both sides. But without the support and the luxury of classroom assistants, disabled children failed too often to gain their teacher's attention. In a class of 40 pupils Sally, a child no-one expected to succeed, rarely got one-to-one tuition. She had been reading well long before she went to school, but now had very few opportunities to shine. The school was a beacon of good intention, but unable to fulfil her aspirations.

At the end of the first school year, Sally's friends moved

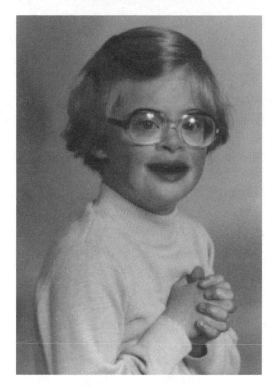

First school photo

to the next class but she stayed in reception. The process was repeated the following year, too. So she lost her friends and had to start all over again with new and younger children. For Sally and her parents time appeared to be standing still. Yet that was to be the least of their worries.

* * * * *

Sally, now almost seven, yearned for promotion after languishing for two years in reception. Just one step-up would have eased her frustration at being left behind with the tiny tots again, feeling like a mother hen with new chicks. It made her quite angry.

"It's not fair," she told Sheila. "I'm beginning to feel ancient, like a mum to the others, helping them with their reading, taking care of them. Then they move up a class, leaving me still here for the next lot to arrive. Why?"

Ken and Sheila couldn't answer, relying on encouraging Sally to be patient; that surely she was now ready to move into the next grade.

It was step-up time for her schoolmates in reception that September and Sally was confident and ready to move up a class with them. But then a real step, only ten inches high and made of hard Yorkshire stone, suddenly shattered her dreams of progress – in fact her future at the village school.

It was the step in the doorway of the second year classroom. The headmaster clearly wanted Sally to progress from reception. He felt she was ready, but someone on high in the education department made an over-riding decision as hard and as cold as that stone step.

Whoever it was decided it wouldn't be safe for Sally, still in her callipers, to try to climb the step. It was too high and dangerous for her, but not the others, moving from the reception class, all two years younger.

At first Sheila was convinced that it was a feeble, unconvincing excuse. She was stunned and angry when the headmaster called her into his office to explain and apologise. "I'm so sorry, Sally cannot remain with us." And then stumbling for words he explained the education authority would be responsible if anything happened to her.

Angry and almost in tears Sheila argued; "It's so unfair. It'll break Sally's heart. She was so excited about moving forward. She's coping so well too; ready to make more progress. Please… let her stay with her friends."

The headmaster shook his head. The decision came from above. "There's nothing I can do. I know it is only a single step, but they feel it could be dangerous for Sally to use it. She could have a nasty fall and we can't take the risk."

Sheila reminded him that two years earlier he had agreed Sally should live her life to the full, whatever the consequences or the risks in the classroom or playground.

"She needs her school and her friends and the same chances as everyone else," said Sheila. "That's all we ask. She'll cope well enough. She'll be careful. She'll climb that step on her hands and knees if she has to, or on her bottom, to stay here…"

It seemed like the end of the world for Sally as she and Sheila trudged home in tears in the rain.

For Sheila and Ken it was a painful reminder of the day they had to tell Sally there would be no more horse riding or visits to the swimming pool. She was only four then and inconsolable for days.

Now she was aware of choices in life, the basics that a village primary school offers; and she wanted to keep them all: the learning and challenges, friends, fun and games in the playground, singing together, nativity plays. They were everything she now treasured so dearly – gone, taken away suddenly. She couldn't believe it could happen like this. Why?

Sheila tried to explain the situation and to reverse the decision, but in the end she was forced to accept it. Now the challenge was to find some way to convince Sally the rejection was only a temporary setback, that she must never give up believing she would become a schoolgirl again. That all her hopes and dreams were still permissible; that there was a way and somehow they would find it.

It didn't take long to come up with the only practical solution. Sheila decided to make their cottage Sally's new classroom, temporarily she hoped.

The big problem was persuading Sally that it would be fun, as good and maybe even better than playing mother hen to the tiny tots in reception.

Sheila's new and flexible curriculum was worked out that weekend. On the Monday, as the village children flocked to school, Sally was too upset to eat her breakfast. She wept buckets as she stood outside Ebor Cottage listening to the school bell ringing out. Inside their cosy two-up, two-down

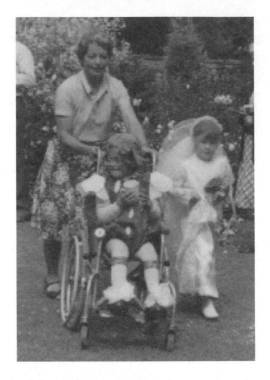

*Sheila, Sally in prizewinning fancy dress as a strawberry,
and her friend Tricia Hodgson.*

terraced home, Sheila mentally prepared her tactics to try
to bring some cheer back into their lives.

It was a grey, rainy Monday and that didn't help as Sheila
put her persuasive powers to the test on her broken-hearted
daughter.

A long, warm cuddle helped a little. It always does at
any age, but Sally wasn't even prepared to return her mum's
comforting smile that all would soon be well.

"Tell you what! We can start this morning with a long
walk," said Sheila. "We'll do some nature studies. It would
be fun. You'd like that wouldn't you?"

Sally wrinkled her nose. "It's raining," she moaned. "I
want to be in school with my friends."

"We'll do some baking," said Sheila, trying to sound inspired and wondering if she had enough flour in the cup-
board. "We could make all sorts of good things, biscuits,

cakes, gingerbread men. And we'll have a party for all your friends after school. They can come any time, every day if you like."

The thought had some appeal and brought a smile and a question; "I will be able to go back to school one day... won't I? I'm not going to have to stay at home all my life?"

"Of course not, darling," said Sheila. "And that's a promise, but until we can sort everything out we must do some work here at home, together. So you will be ready when the time comes... It will be fun. That's another promise."

As the days and weeks drifted into months Sally never ever lost faith in her mother's promises.

Sheila and Ken soon realised their daughter was too strong-willed to give up hope on anything, especially herself or her dreams of returning to the classroom.

It was to take two long years.

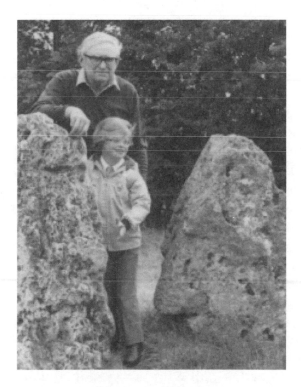

Ken and Sally in the Cotswolds

8

Welburn Hall welcome

The next two years were difficult for the Johnsons. Sally got her home teacher, but only for one hour a day, mostly for English lessons. It wasn't long enough for an inquisitive child keen to learn. Sheila, who desperately wanted to be mother to Sally, not her teacher, found herself forced into the role. When Jean Healey, her home teacher, left half-way through the morning, Sheila continued to teach Sally other subjects, including nature studies. At the end of the first year, there was barely a stone in the village they had not turned over in search of creepy-crawlies or whatever was underneath; or a museum for miles around they had not visited. The pace continued with endless sessions sticking things together with glue to create puppets and other weird and wonderful things.

Sheila's inventiveness was stretched to maintain Sally's interest. But for a small child, half the fun of learning is having someone to share the experience. Sally's great love was her Cavalier King Charles spaniel, Becky, but she desperately missed her friends. Her opportunities for socialising were governed by the school bell. As it rang out for home time, she would sit in the front window eagerly awaiting friends she had asked to tea and to play. To their great credit, they never failed to arrive.

Sally was able to join the village Brownie group, revelling in the comradeship it gave her. She proudly made her Brownie Promise without even a single prompt, and was awarded 13 badges, all with no special allowances for her disability. These experiences offered some brief snatches of life she so desperately wanted – but they were not enough for a girl with such an extravagant hunger to be like others.

One test for a Brownie badge was to cook sausages after pricking them with a skewer. She amused the rest of the Brownie pack and examiner by turning it into an hilarious mock operation. She pretended to be a surgeon, telling each sausage: "This is quite painless, so be brave."

Suddenly that proverbial light in the tunnel appeared. A visit to nearby Welburn Hall, a school for children with physical disabilities, convinced Sheila it was the ideal place for Sally. The school had never accepted a child with Down's Syndrome and the education authority was reluctant to admit a pupil with what was perceived as a "learning disability", no matter how high her IQ. Jean Healey, Sally's excellent home teacher, became determined to help progress Sally's education and promise. After persistent lobbying, Jean obtained consent to take Sally to Welburn Hall's hydrotherapy pool for weekly exercise sessions. It helped to open a door. Sally's heart specialist, Dr Olive Scott, wrote to the authority saying the hydrotherapy was also essential to help with Sally's physical problems. The education officials were persuaded. After two frustrating years of exclusion, Sally was a schoolgirl once more, out in the world, making new friends. She was elated.

She travelled the 12 miles to school every day in the care of Mike Eccles, a friendly taxi driver who loved Country and Western music. His enthusiasm for it was infectious and the pair spent the daily journey singing their favourites with gusto. In the classroom Sally was also full of enthusiasm. After two anxious years she eagerly immersed herself in everything Welburn Hall had to offer.

She made friends with a boy called James Ferry, who had cerebral palsy and shared her lively sense of humour. They plotted to make life more interesting for themselves and their teachers.

Each weekend, Sally would seek out difficult spellings

to include in her news report. On Monday morning in class she and James would struggle to keep straight faces as Sally innocently asked how to spell "iridescent", "paraphernalia", or equally testing words. They were delighted when the teacher had to reach for a dictionary but it was not always one-sided, however. Despite her impressive vocabulary, Sally made the occasional but memorable gaffe. She was frequently reminded of one when she called a poppadom a condom.

One factor that defied change for the better was Sally's intense dislike of maths. Her health was still fragile and she frequently experienced dizzy spells that required attention from the school nurse. Surprise, surprise! These attacks often occurred during maths, conveniently giving Sally an escape from those baffling numbers.

Sheila's relationship with Sally continued to blossom in a special way. The periods they spent apart made their quality time together more enjoyable. They could have more fun together. Sally's enthusiasm for learning, apart from maths, brought its own rewards. When she was eight she entered a poetry competition to win a coveted Blue Peter badge from her favourite BBC television programme. It was dedicated to her beloved pet Becky.

> I have a little Cavalier
> She's brown and white and very dear
> With one big spot upon her head
> A mark of breeding so it's said.
>
> If I'm not well she stays with me
> And often climbs onto my knee.
> I never feel alone with her
> And love to stroke her silky fur.

Sally was now making remarkable progress, fully justifying her acceptance as a half-day pupil at Welburn Hall and the excellent care and tuition it offered. She was there until she was 17 and before leaving she won a Duke of Edinburgh's bronze award. She was unable to go on for a silver or gold because there was no allowance for her disability.

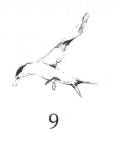

9

Gift brings TV fame

Christmas is a magical experience in Thornton-le-Dale, for everyone, of any age; and especially for those who visit to share the joy. The village overflows with history, charm and warmth all year round. It may not be a Brigadoon, shrouded in moorland mist and mystery, but at Christmas it can be enchanting.

Thornton-le-Dale, with its fast-flowing stream snaking and gurgling around stone cottages, was once voted the most beautiful in Yorkshire against stiff competition. Pictures of its famous thatched cottage, village cross and stocks are exported around the world on postcards, biscuit tins and chocolate boxes.

All around the village is the England foreign tourists expect to see: lush forests where wild deer roam and bashful badgers hide, purple heathered moorland, ancient abbeys and castles, quaint fishing villages, market towns... and all the good and charm the lovely district of Ryedale, North Yorkshire and its people, can offer.

Legend says Robin Hood was born at nearby Hartoft village and hid in the Saxon crypt at Lastingham with Much the miller's son after being unjustly branded outlaws. That was about 700 years before Victorian "penny-dreadful" writers kidnapped the legendary Yorkshire hero and planted him in Nottinghamshire.

Sally, born in Scarborough Hospital Maternity Ward on June 28th 1974 at midday, loved her village. It offered everything a child could wish for – and more. And the village folk learned to love Sally.

She was now a happy teenager but she had no idea Christmas 1991 would gift her a special talent, a deep love of art that had filled her parents' lives with so much joy and satisfaction.

Secretly Ken spent weeks making Sally a wooden artist's box and he and Sheila filled it with watercolour paints, brushes and a sketching pad.

Somehow Sally always refused to say what she would like for Christmas. Her response was "Surprise me! I love surprises."

After all the hugs and kisses on that Christmas morning the response to her surprise gift was "Fantastic! When can we start painting together? Now... please..."

Ken tried to conceal how much her enthusiasm meant to him. "Let's have breakfast first before you get your first lesson," he grinned.

Over the years Ken had delighted in the close, loving bond Sheila and Sally had developed. They had become like sisters. Now, perhaps, painting pictures would bring him as close to his daughter.

Soon after breakfast they sat together, Ken explaining and encouraging, but Sally impatient to make a start. He showed her how to sketch and shape a picture in pencil, how to mix watercolour paints and apply them. Sally soon grasped the basic techniques of light and shade to bring her work alive.

Her first painting was a view of the nearby village of Hovingham. Ken was impressed and Sally delighted with his praise. She took the picture to Welburn Hall to show her teacher what she had created during her Christmas holiday.

"Can I buy your picture, Sally?" her teacher asked.

Sally was delighted. Being an artist's daughter she couldn't wait to get home to impress Ken with the crisp £5 note from her first sale.

"You've sold more than me today!" Ken protested, feigning a slight resentment. Sally was ecstatic and eager to learn

how to perfect her tone values, so important in all paintings.

One night after dinner as they sat around the television
watching the news, Sally saw heart-rending pictures of a
starving baby wailing pitifully in the heat of an African
drought. Her tears flowed for the images of emaciated
people trapped in helplessness and despair.

"I'm going to send that baby my £5." Sally announced.
"Then I'm going to paint and paint and sell lots of pictures
... and send the money to help them!"

Her parents smiled at her good intentions. Little did they
realise how Sally's gesture would involve her painting
about 2,500 original watercolours to raise more than
£250,000 (including all reproductions) for good causes over
nine years.

Sally was true to her mission in life. Every original picture was sold immediately with a long waiting list. Word
of her artistic talent and charity campaign spread eventually world-wide.

Sally quickly became the talk of the district. "She's disabled,
you know," they said. "Down's Syndrome. Oh, but she's a
grand lass ... lovely pictures ... make a nice present ..."

Among the Christmas cards Sheila sent out in 1991 was
one to former neighbours Liz and Bill Gabbitas living on
the Algarve. "Sally has taken up painting," Sheila wrote.
"She sells them and gives all the money she makes to charities." Impressed by Sally's crusade, they mentioned it to
Amanda, their daughter, a BBC children's television producer. She phoned Sally to find out more.

"I would like you to tell your story for viewers," Amanda
said. "It would help people to understand about Down's
Syndrome."

She wanted Sally for the starring role in a special feature
called *All About Me* on the BBC's *Going Live*, a prime-time
Saturday morning series for children.

Days later a television crew arrived in the village to film
her story unaware Sally was about to have an attack of

nerves. She came down to breakfast in her nightie to plead: "I don't feel very well." She disappeared upstairs where Sheila found her sobbing on the bed, overwhelmed by the occasion. She was only suffering from her first bout of stage fright, something she quickly mastered. The TV crew had no idea of the drama in the bedroom as they set up their camera, lights and sound boom.

"Oh, Sally," Sheila said. "They have come all the way from London to film, you can't let them down now."

"I can't do it," Sally said, shaking her head. "I won't be very good."

"You will. You've never failed to meet a challenge. This is probably one of the biggest you'll ever have to face," urged Sheila.

They knelt together and prayed for courage. Within minutes Sally leapt to her feet and with thumbs up said, "I'm ready. I can do it!"

By 9.00 a.m. on that bitter January morning, Sally sat in front of the camera, sketching a village scene with Ken and talking through chattering teeth. She was a natural. No one had to tell her what to say. She talked about her life, her voluntary work with the elderly and infirm and her painting. Sally told viewers, "I have Down's Syndrome but that doesn't mean people should pity me or others like me. I enjoy my life." Two days later the delighted Amanda and her television crew left after filming on the moors, at Welburn Hall school and a care home for the elderly. At the end of the film Sally was asked what she felt was most important in life. Her reply intensely moved the crew and later millions of viewers. "To be happy," she said. "And to make others happy."

Ten days later the 10-minute long film was screened and something remarkable happened. Hundreds of phone calls and letters poured into the BBC from doctors, care workers, teachers and health visitors all over the country, all expressing interest and delight in Sally's story. They asked if they could buy a copy of the film to inspire and encourage others. Teenagers wrote about the problems and frustrations in their lives and how Sally's story had helped them to face up to them. Many calls came from parents of Down's Syndrome children, inspired by Sally's achievements. Some became pen-friends for life. Orders for paintings came from around the world, keeping Sally busy for months. When the BBC screened the film a second time two years later the response was even greater. In ten minutes Sally had changed attitudes and lives and it was only the beginning.

10

Breaking down barriers

For a little while the tide of Sally's fortunes and talents flowed smoothly. She won a national painting competition run by Mencap to design a Christmas card, which attracted thousands of entries from children and adults. Her success aroused the interest of the Down's Syndrome Association, who asked if she would paint some pictures for them. The arrangement became a life-long link. For many years Sally designed the Association's Christmas card, and she produced 12 paintings for its silver anniversary calendar, a big seller. A windswept moorland scene was used for the charity's national awareness poster campaign, giving Sally a real surprise when she saw it splashed across a bus shelter, just one of thousands nationwide. It was even displayed on the walls of escalators at London tube stations. The poster said simply: "This is the work of Sally Johnson. She's sold more paintings than Van Gogh. She also just happens to have Down's Syndrome."

The association saw Sally as a natural ambassador to promote awareness of their work. It sent a painting to the Prime Minister, and he was so impressed he wrote to her personally. In his letter, John Major said her picture, hanging in his office at Number 10, expressed "the peace and tranquillity missing from my busy life".

Scores of letters arrived each week for Sally but she dealt with her new-found fame and fan mail in the same calm, self-effacing way that she dealt with disappointments in her life. Success and praise somehow seemed to pass her by.

She was delighted because of what it meant to those she was determined to help. Orders meant paintings and money for charities. Every penny went to good causes.

Sally's paintings became her life work. She would do about five originals a week and sell them instantly. Ken and Sally were thrilled when they were invited to exhibit their paintings in a working watermill, a popular attraction on the River Esk at Danby near Whitby. For weeks they painted frantically together and Sally managed to produce 35 watercolours. With Sheila busy cutting mounts, framing and labelling them their home took on the air of a cottage industry.

The exhibition opened on Good Friday and people came from all over the UK to see their paintings and to meet Sally, Ken and Sheila. Before the Bank Holiday weekend was over every one of Sally's pictures had been sold. It created a problem because the exhibition had seven more months to run.

"We'll just have to paint some more," piped Sally, enthusiastic as ever. She produced at least seven paintings each week to keep the show alive and continued selling her work at the mill for the next five years. She also displayed her paintings in the Tea Garden restaurant in nearby Malton Market Place where hundreds of originals and prints were sold.

With each brushstroke Sally was breaking down social barriers facing her and others like her, proving they had skills and talents to offer. Her success resulted in numerous stories which appeared in the local and national press and magazines. Each article meant a renewed demand for original paintings and prints.

Tom Petrie, the *Sunday People*'s "Man of the People" columnist told readers about her. His Editor sent Sally a cheque for £500 to buy more painting materials. She decided, with his permission, to distribute it to charities instead.

As demand for Sally's watercolours became so great the Down's Syndrome Association produced prints of her finest work. They also appeared on T-shirts and notelets, still a best-selling fundraiser. Changing people's attitudes was one thing; altering society's view as a whole was more difficult. Despite all her achievements, Sally was still not allowed to open a bank account in her own name because of her perceived "learning difficulties", that politically-correct label for the mentally disabled. Sheila and Ken eventually managed to get special permission for Sally to open a Halifax Building Society account. All the monies she received were paid into it. The only withdrawals were for her art materials. Sally would only have to catch a glimpse of a disaster or urgent appeal on the news to consult her Halifax balance to see how much she could send to help.

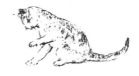

11

Winning hearts and minds

Most people who met Sally and bought her pictures had no idea how ill she was. They saw her callipers and her wheel-chair. They knew about Down's Syndrome, if only vaguely. What they could not see, and what Sally never spoke of, was her pain and suffering as she painted.

As a child she was never well enough to spend a full day at school. The morning sessions left her so exhausted she needed the afternoons to rest. By her mid-teens, Sally's dam-aged heart had become so enlarged that her spine began to twist, pushing one hip higher than the other. This caused her to walk with a rolling gait. She also developed severe gout in her joints which, on bad days, made the slightest movement agony. She collapsed, sometimes several times a day, and would turn an alarming shade of blue. She would smile afterwards and say, "I've had another one of my do's… that's all. I'm OK now." Sheila and Ken were aware that their daughter's health was deteriorating and nothing could be done to help her. Somehow she kept going, often to the point of exhaustion. Sally was determined to paint pictures and live her life to the full.

Armed with Ordnance Survey maps they discovered for-gotten and hidden places – fords, packhorse bridges and brooks – where they could take Sally to sketch undisturbed. Often, she had to break off to rest in the family's old caravanette, but when they left a location she would have the vital sketches for her new paintings.

Ken and Sheila were amazed at her tenacity. No matter

how ill she felt she never complained.

During these spells of desperate illness Sally refused to stay in bed, determined to seize every moment of the life she was given, and achieve some good from it. Inspired by her courage, Ken and Sheila made a pledge. If Sally could live life at that incredible pace, then so could they. Every day had a plan. They would decide where to go and what they wanted to do and defy all obstacles to achieve it.

12

Evergreen tribe

Sally's most endearing quality, rarely found in the young today, was a natural rapport with the elderly. She delighted in their company but who could resist her natural charm and enthusiasm to bond together in friendship?

Those who witnessed this say Sally appeared to focus on the individual underneath, their soul perhaps, in a remarkable way. She could demolish barriers with what they describe as an amazing X-ray vision. Maybe it was because she never appeared to notice signs of ageing or its effect on the body and mind.

Sheila's mother was a great influence on Sally, more than simply her Gran. She was a special friend with a fund of stories, real and fairy-tale, exciting but mostly funny. Gran believed laughter was good medicine for problems, if not a cure.

Life hadn't always been kind for Gran, who was born in 1903. She never grumbled, always content and thankful for the good things in her hard and sad life during and between two terrible world wars. "Counting my blessings," she would say. "There are so many others worse off."

Like so many of her generation she had struggled to raise Sheila and Pat against all the odds. Somehow she managed to gift them her compassion for the old and disabled. You could say it was in Sally's genes.

So it was natural for Sally to have a burning desire to do her bit for humanity. She decided to focus on the elderly with age-related health problems. She was in her last year at Welburn Hall and volunteered for work experience at the council-run residential home for the elderly in Whitby Road, Pickering.

This also gave her the opportunity to fulfil the community service part of the tasks required to win a Duke of Edinburgh's bronze award.

She also completed a detailed survey on access for the disabled in various parts of the Ryedale District, another task for the bronze award. It was achieved in a practical manner from the wheelchair she had to rely on to get around. Curiously it was the alternative task to taking a long walk which she was physically incapable of doing. She repeated her access probe as a task for the Gateway Gold some years later. The two studies spurred local businesses and Councillors to implement her suggestions to help the disabled in Ryedale towns and villages.

At 17, her Welburn Hall school days almost over, Sally quickly found an exciting if new challenge. She set out to inspire and lift the spirits of a group of elderly people who, through failing health, had lost interest in life.

She volunteered to work one day a week, in whatever way her schedule and imagination could devise, at Evergreen, a private care home in Scarborough. It cared for around 20 residents with Alzheimer's or age-related dementia.

Sheila drove Sally there each week, and on the journey home and late into evening they discussed the problems and challenges and how to overcome them. The residents appeared to have lost the will to do anything but doze away their days, or stare blankly at the TV screen.

As a teacher Sheila knew how to stimulate backward children and she and Sally were soon bouncing ideas around. But would they work with the Evergreen residents? There was a need to get them talking, about their lives and what had interested and influenced them. "Everyone has a story to tell, like Gran," said Sally. "If I can get them talking about themselves it would be a start. I need to get to know everyone by name and their life stories." So her research began into early twentieth-century history and entertainment, like the music halls and early radio; its stars, comedians, singers and songs. It wasn't difficult to find some old records that hadn't been played for decades and put them onto tape. "To get them talking I need to know all about those early days," she wrote in her diary. "I want to help them re-live happier times."

Sally dipped into her charity funds for ingredients to make cakes and biscuits and peppermint creams, the sort Gran and Sheila had taught her to bake.

At Evergreen Sally quickly broke the ice with her tasty treats and music. Soon a singalong was a regular feature of her visits and between songs memories came flooding out to Sally.

Soon everyone looked forward to her visits. "Their eyes light up when she arrives," said Maureen Middleton, owner of Evergreen. "She was a ray of sunshine, a special friend. They loved her so much."

"Gosh! There's a great book in their stories," Sally enthused as she jotted them down in her diary. "One saw a Zeppelin crash in World War One. Exciting! So many happy memories; but also some sad. I'd like to include them in my book when I write it… one day I will."

Every Easter Sally organised a special party with chocolate eggs for everyone as they put on their Easter bonnets she helped them to make.

She directed a cabaret with residents each doing a turn, singing, often a song from their childhood days, or a recitation memorised for school or their church anniversary. Impromptu pantomimes were on the social menu at Christmas.

Sally devised a special show, adapted from a picture book by Susan Jeffers, of Henry Wadsworth Longfellow's *Hiawatha*. Everyone was given a role, one of the tribe or animals in the story.

"There's no business like show business," Sally sang to them.

It wasn't just vanity that made Sally choose the starring

role of Nokomis, Daughter of the Moon, for herself. It was necessary to provide the lead to create the mood from start to finish. She was producer, director, choreographer and music director and, of course, the star.

She got rave notices from the rest of her cast at Evergreen for make-up and costume and, most of all, for her clear delivery of Longfellow's immortal lines to the accompaniment of a drum beat, starting with:

> By the shores of Gitche Gumee,
> By the shining big-sea-water,
> Stood the wigwam of Nokomis,
> Daughter of the Moon, Nokomis.

It was more than a loving oration. Sally had also created a musical with her range of electronic musical instruments placed in the hands of the Evergreen tribe who responded with great enthusiasm and near perfect timing to her coaching.

At times Sally dipped into her painting charity fund to treat residents to a cream tea in a café or a day at the chalet a friend had rented for them overlooking Scarborough beach.

Sally was full of happy surprises, but the Evergreen tribe sprang a special one for her on her 18th birthday.

That morning as she looked out of her bedroom window she spotted a minibus, festooned with balloons and streamers, rounding the corner. It stopped outside Ebor Cottage and an Evergreen chorus sang "Happy birthday … dear Sally …"

In the minibus was a well-stocked picnic hamper and simple presents which helped to make Sally's majority one of her most cherished birthdays.

Over seven years, until she was too ill to travel, she made her weekly trips to Evergreen to talk, listen and entertain, always with imaginative ideas and love.

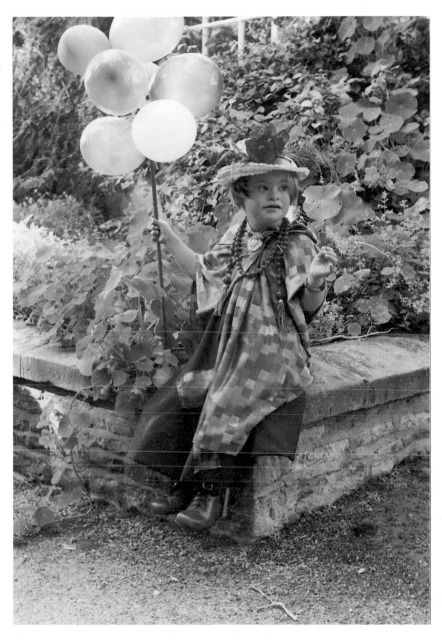

Sally, the balloon seller

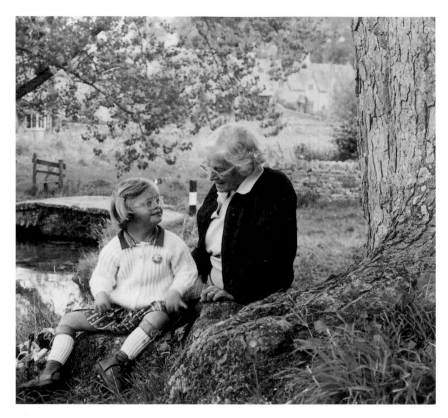

Chat with Gran

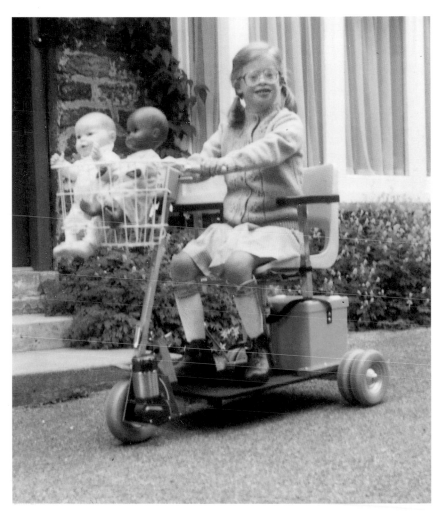

Sally scooting with her 'family', Peter and Sam

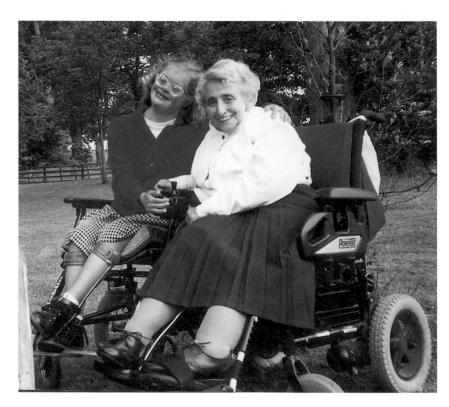

Wheelchair fellowship with Auntie Pat

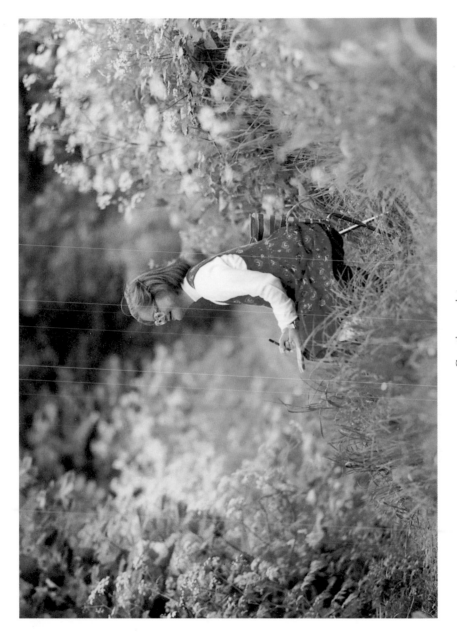

Creating a picture

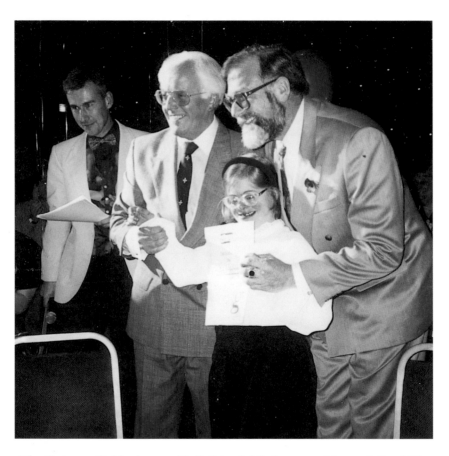

The Gateway Gold winner with (left to right) Compere, Mencap's Lord Rix
and Gateway Club Chairman Roger Galletley

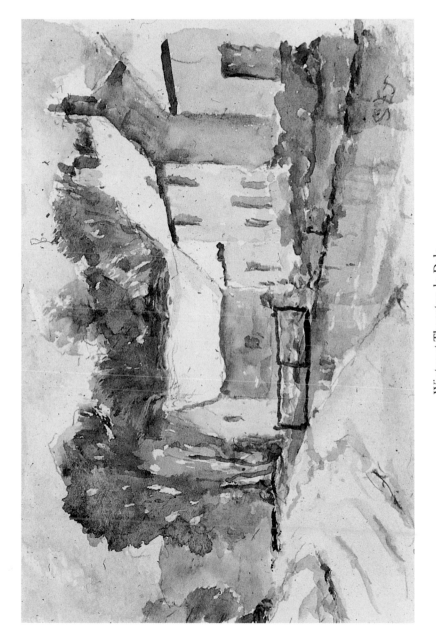

Winter at Thornton-le-Dale

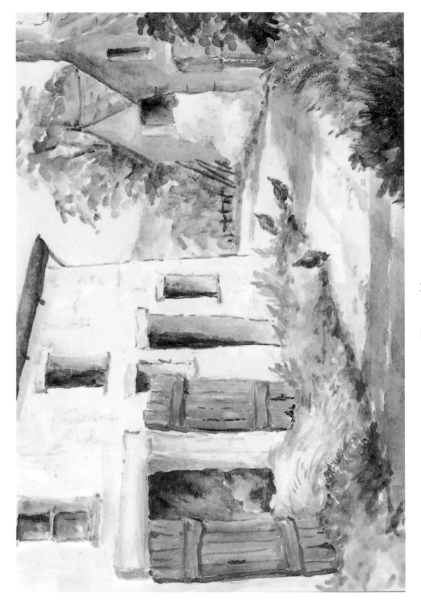

Hen-pecking

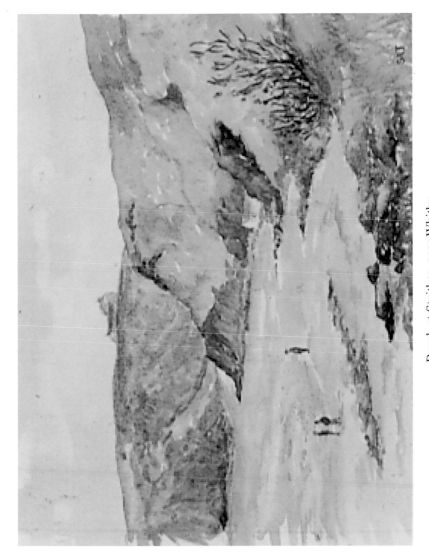

Beach at Staithes, near Whitby

9

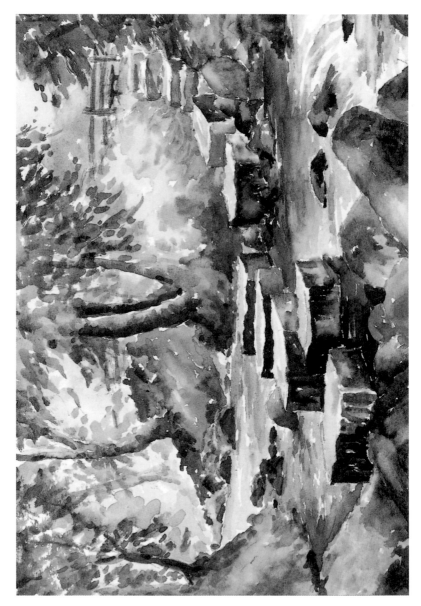

Stepping stones at Beckhole

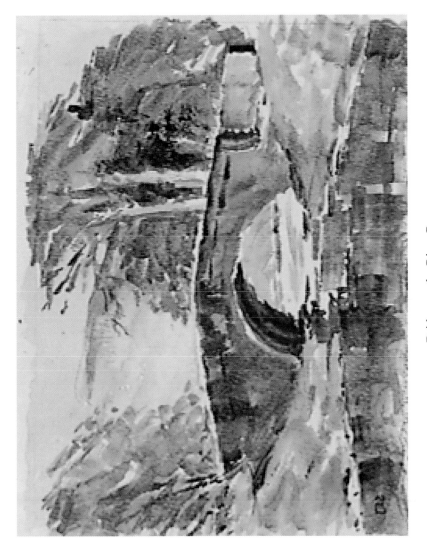

Bridge on the River Rye

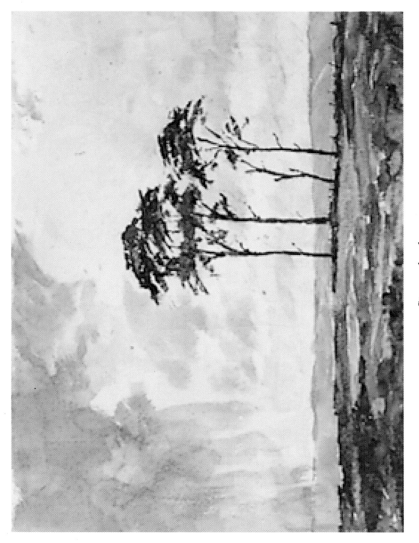

Storm clouds

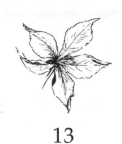

13

Bronze to Silver

For Sally the years at Welburn Hall were sheer bliss, her idea of joyful independence; and leaving was a sad and difficult time. Suddenly, after almost eight years, she was anchored back at home, living in a frustrating void, desperately seeking to fill her time.

Her whole life so far had been a challenge – just to stay alive. Now she yearned for a new challenge, something exciting … fun.

At 18 most teenagers are busy earning a living; or off to university. A few, the more adventurous, are planning a gap year, backpacking somewhere around the world or doing good works .

Sally's serious health problems, and also being classified as "special needs", meant she was unemployable. Of course she had her painting, which she loved. It had become her life mission to sell her work to raise money for local and national charities. It was almost full-time, but no longer a challenge for a young lady determined to increase and balance out her interests – and make new friends too!

Her social life had depended so much on Welburn Hall and school friends who came from a wide area of Britain. All she could do now was to try to keep in touch with them, but, like Sally, they had their own problems and challenges.

The Cauwood Day Centre offered Sally a way forward with courses in pottery and other craftwork. It lifted her spirits for several months but she still craved for that special personal challenge. Then suddenly what she had hoped and prayed for was on offer.

Sally worked hard to win her Duke of Edinburgh's bronze award, which proved a true test of her natural intelligence and will to win. Her major achievement among the many qualifying tasks was a detailed report on lack of access for the disabled in Ryedale.

The disappointment for Sally was that silver and gold awards were not open to those with special needs who had achieved the bronze. Of course there was no way they could even attempt the demanding physical tasks involved in those higher awards.

However, there was a new challenge open to Sally and others like her. It was inspired by the Duke of Edinburgh's Awards, adapted and devised by Millie Lewis for Mencap and called The Gateway Awards, bronze, silver and gold. Sally, who had already qualified for bronze with the Duke of Edinburgh's scheme, entered for the silver.

The Gateway challenges are a test of self-reliance, courage and staying power spread over a period of eighteen months for the silver with a further two years for the gold.

As they studied the details Sheila warned, "This is really tough, Sally. It's not going to be a flash in the pan. It will demand patience, careful study – and lots of determination. Do you think you could do it?" She was really concerned about Sally's failing health.

"It's just what I need," said Sally. "I can do it! Let's go!"

The first real test of Sally's courage and determination was to learn to swim, the only physical challenge she could attempt for the Gateway Silver award.

She had to swim as far as she could, even if only a short distance. Sally completed six lengths of the Scarborough swimming pool, despite severe heart-related chest pains. This was a particular achievement for Sally as she had been forced to give up swimming as a toddler on medical advice, although she had loved it even then, scaring her parents by doggy-paddling into the deep end wearing inflatable armbands.

Sally was a well-travelled child around the most attractive rural parts of England, searching, with her parents, for scenes to paint. So her study of map reading, to basic army standards, became just an additional exercise during painting expeditions, especially in the North Yorkshire Dales. Her most favourite place, Dent Dale, can seem like a trip into another century. The village of Dent with its cobbled streets, stone cottages and the narrow road alongside the fast-flowing River Dee is an artist's dream. Frequent holidays there, in a static caravan on a local farm, gave Sally the opportunity to concentrate on the more creative elements of the Gateway Challenge.

Her relationship with her parents was always close but casual and, in fact, from her early teens Sally always called them Ken and Sheila.

Ken helped Sally acquire a keen eye for selecting and framing a scene for her paintings. It proved useful when she had to take photographs to illustrate the reports she wrote for the judges after completing a Gateway challenge.

Her love of nature also gave her a head start to the longest-running challenge: identifying, recording and pressing wild flowers as they appeared over a full year, starting with snow drops, with a whole colourful flurry to follow.

One of her greatest older friends in the village was Miss Maurine Bawden, a retired primary school teacher in her eighties, a keen student of wild flowers and an excellent photographer. Maurine was delighted to offer advice on her hobbies to assist Sally's quest for the silver Gateway Challenge.

The Gateway judges were impressed with the imaginative and artistic way Sally used her pressed flowers to decorate candles, bookmarks and even lampshades, a talent taught and encouraged by Sheila.

Every challenge for the silver award was completed on time, supervised and encouraged by Sandra Ward at the Pickering Gateway Club. It is run at the Wilf Ward Family Trust's Isabella Court, a respite and also a social centre for young people with learning disabilities.

Wilf Ward (at the time of writing, 86 years of age) is a remarkable former Yorkshire farmer. He and his late brother, Frank, used their engineering skills to create a successful business in Ryedale. When he retired he invested most of his fortune to set up a charity devoted to helping people trapped in disability. He also wanted to become involved, and is still active as Chairman of the Trust, seeing his investment give the disabled a focus in life, hope, fellowship and social opportunities.

It was at the local Gateway Club that Sally made many friends, like Ben Moss who gave a very caring friendship that lasted a lifetime.

Wilf Ward found Sally's courage and certain charisma an inspiration to others. He was delighted to be asked to present her with her silver award. She was the first to win it and now, even with her increasing health problems, she was determined to go for gold.

14

Healing with music

To everyone Sally was always the happy extrovert who kept her pain to herself, never ever complaining. To the outside world she gave the impression all was well in her life. She learned to laugh at life and herself from a very early age. For Sally laughter was good medicine for the unbearable.

But it was the soothing value of good music that helped her to forget, if only briefly at times, the pain and discomfort of a serious heart defect, gout, myopia and a permanent shortage of oxygen in the blood. Before she was one year old she danced in her baby-bouncer to the rhythm of music played on a gramophone, a gift, with lots of lively records, from her Great Aunt Doris.

Family friends Bill and Liz Gabbitas, who lived in the village, also proved a powerful influence on Sally when she was very young, taking a great interest in her progress. It was their daughter, Amanda, a BBC children's programme producer, who brought the teenage Sally's story onto television to inspire millions around the world.

When Bill and Liz went to live in Portugal they also gave Sally, then only five, an electric organ to make her own music in her bedroom. Over the years Ken and Sheila bought her an electric keyboard, a guitar, violin, drum kit, a range of percussion instruments – even a mouth organ when she was only seven. Sally loved to play Happy Birthday down the phone to friends and family. By the age of ten she had developed a serious (for her age) taste in music, ranging from the lighter Beethoven to The Beatles. She also developed a love for Mozart, Chopin and Tchaikovsky, especially his ballet music, which she tried to dance to. She also read everything she could about her favourite composers and pop stars. Cliff Richard was always her number one.

It was Cliff and also The Beatles who gave her the urge to write lyrics and compose music – to get more involved in a creative way. Music was also greatly valued as a therapy for the disabled pupils at Welburn Hall. It was something Sally missed when, almost 18, she had to leave the Hall for what was another uncertain period in her life. She called it her doldrums and felt lost and frustrated for a while but, true to form, she bounced back.

Sheila says: "Sally would have made a very good actress, especially in comedy. She could be so witty at any time which endeared her to everyone. Even when her life seemed to hit a really bad patch, which was too often, she always felt sure something good was about to happen for her. She had such great faith."

Something new and exciting developed the day Raymond and Mary Abbotson came into her life. They not only taught her how to expand her interest in music but also how she could use it to help others.

The Abbotsons are music therapists, renowned world-wide for their research and work, especially among youngsters with a wide range of disabilities. They call it "healing with music". Now elderly and semi-retired they have a consultancy at the University of York and provide information and advice for the growing global interest in music therapy.

In the Western world music therapy is mostly provided in clinics for children. In their early pioneering years Raymond and Mary delivered it to the disabled from their van full of electronic equipment which they designed themselves, plus a piano. It was a fun way, with immediate appeal for the young while creating a valuable service in rural North Yorkshire.

The Abbotson Trust for Music Therapy came into being

in the tiny hamlet of Kirby Mills, Kirkbymoorside, where they still maintain an open-house "think-tank" for music therapists and health care professionals.

They describe their work as, simply, "to offer music therapy to help people develop their potential, improve the quality of life and promote healthy change". Their work brought them and Sally together in a deep, long-lasting friendship and her story is a fascinating case history available for others to study.

The Abbotsons believe music is a God-given gift to soothe, entertain and help anyone at any age with disabilities, even the frail and elderly and adult psychiatric patients.

Can there be any doubts whatsoever about the deep, often overwhelming feelings of joy music provides or the memories and emotions it arouses?

The *Concise Oxford Dictionary of Quotations* says it all, in cryptic comment or verse, mostly in praise of music therapy. Victorian poet Robert Browning asked: "Is music sent up to God?" John Dryden, a 17th-century poet, wrote: "music shall untune the sky". Even playwright Noel Coward wrote a line of dialogue: "strange how potent cheap music is". In *Twelfth Night* Shakespeare wrote the immortal line: "If music be the food of love play on ..."

This all explains why we are moved to sadness or joy by music of all kinds; although we rarely wonder how the first musical sounds were created by primitive man. No doubt by accident! Or the way it has developed over thousands of years from the celestial to something called Rap or Hip-Hop, which seems to have its great appeal among the young.

The Abbotsons say Sally was more a pupil than a patient. "She proved to be a most interesting young person with unusual gifts," says Mary. "Her parents shared artistic and professional skills. This enabled them to nurture Sally's natural talents to the full."

At the time Sally wore spectacles with thick lenses, had leg supports, a serious heart condition and other health problems, according to the Abbotsons' case report.

"She was quickly into three-part improvisations playing drum and cymbal followed over the following two years by creating musical pictures on a range of percussion instruments and at the piano," says Mary. "We challenged Sally's learning abilities by introducing songs or music which demanded precise timing at exact points. They were not easy but she always showed great determination to master difficulties."

The Abbotson influence was later reflected in Sally's own work among the elderly with Alzheimer's and dementia at the Evergreen Care Home in Scarborough. She used the music therapy skills to persuade the residents to participate and be stimulated.

During an interview Sally had with a BBC Radio York reporter she was asked how she felt about music therapy. Her immediate response was; "It can have an amazing effect. It seems to create a lovely feeling of peace and joy. You should try it for yourself and you'll realise what I mean."

Which says it all without any help from the *Oxford Dictionary of Quotations*.

15

Go for Gold!

Having achieved her Gateway Silver Award Sally, now 19, was surprised to discover she was the only entrant for it and was now also going solo for gold. "If I'm the only runner I'll have to win," she joked, but to Mencap, who had developed the scheme, she was an inspirational standard bearer.

Sally's silver had already inspired others, many older than herself, to enter for the Gateway Bronze, the first hurdle of the new challenge.

Her determination and progress over the three-and-a-half years of silver and gold could be described as a minor miracle. She believed in miracles. She had to because of her constant health problems. The slightest exertion placed great strain on her heart, leaving her breathless and her face turning a worrying shade of blue.

Sheila was a constant companion, with a portable oxygen cylinder to bring Sally round during these emergencies. They often happened several times a day. But after each attack Sally would smile and say: "It's just one of my little do's ... that's all," and insist: "I'm OK. Don't worry."

Sheila, who had her own health problems, was concerned. She also had other family worries. Ken had diabetes and, now in his seventies, suffered a heart attack while on a family painting holiday in Derbyshire. Gran's dementia had worsened and she was now in a nursing home in the village, just a short walk from the Johnson cottage, so the family could visit her every day.

It was to prove a period of sad lows for the family as Sally's health and energy levels began to weaken alarmingly.

After a hospital check-up the specialist had grim news. "I'm afraid Sally has only a very, very short time to live," he emphasised after taking Sheila aside.

He wouldn't put a time on it, which only created a constant anxiety. How long? When? Today, a week, month? Ken and Sheila agonised for days and nights before deciding Sally must never know how short her life might be, not now with the challenge for the Gateway Gold dominating her hopes and dreams.

Irrelevant issues tend to cloud minds in crisis and Sheila began to worry about making any plans involving Sally, even buying new clothes or booking a holiday. Perhaps it was natural, even better, to fret about getting Sally a new, warm winter coat in October than imagine life without her.

Then suddenly the cloud lifted and Ken and Sheila came to the only logical decision – to enjoy each day with her as it came. "It's best. That's all we can do now," said Ken who, despite his serious health problems, was painting again. He even used his engineering skills to make all the components for a 6ft garden telescope and an engine for his bike.

Together they proved, without trying too hard, that faith, love and good humour can conquer despair and ease problems.

Ebor Cottage is one of the oldest in Thornton-le-Dale, with a steep and narrow staircase and climbing it was proving too much for Sally. So, Sheila, weighing only 8st 7lbs, somehow managed to carry her slightly lighter daughter upstairs several times a day. She never made a fuss or sought help, but a family friend, the elderly Miss Maurine Bawden, decided to buy them a Stannah stairlift. Its installation greatly improved the quality of life at Ebor Cottage, giving Sheila's health and Sally's sense of independence more than a big lift at a vital time.

With so many problems weighing heavily on the family

their spirit remained strong. They were determined to do all they could to encourage Sally's bid for gold, which included becoming proficient in first aid and home nursing.

Auntie Pat, a distinguished member of the St John's Ambulance Brigade for around 50 years, was a valuable tutor. She had become an honoured Superintendent after devoting most of her service to training hundreds of cadets in East Yorkshire. Many went on to careers in the National Health Service.

Pat devised all the accident and emergency scenarios for Sally who, while taking them all seriously, managed to create lots of laughs. Family and friends became patients to be examined, placed in the recovery position or resuscitated. Pat, born disabled and wheelchair-bound since an horrific accident later in life, said: "If she could have taken it up Sally would have made a fine nurse. The study of first aid and home nursing is a serious business, but learning how to do it well must also be fun. Laughter can be a great aid to learning the right and wrong ways of doing things. I think most who teach would subscribe to that theory. Sally proved it. She was a brilliant pupil, but hilarious with it."

One year into Sally's Gold challenge Ken suddenly became seriously ill with septicaemia. Sally had to stay with her Auntie Pat in Bridlington while Sheila sat by Ken's bedside watching his life ebb away.

Sally, like her mother, had the firm belief death was not the end; that Ken had gone to a better place. His death brought them even closer together as they visited Gran daily in the nursing home. Her life was also coming to a close. The Gateway gold challenge was, thankfully, a useful diversion from grief and sadness.

Perhaps the most difficult challenge for Sally was learning Makaton, the sign language for those with severe learning difficulties, but she had a sympathetic teacher.

It took Sheila two years to become proficient in Makaton when she was a primary school teacher in London and the Midlands, but her new pupil mastered it in just 18 months.

Some Gateway challenges were long-term; others simpler, like planning and taking a self-catering holiday, preparing meals and shopping, although Sally was unable to carry anything heavy.

Her greatest pleasure was the time she spent with her elderly friends at the Evergreen Care Home in Scarborough, a long-term and essential task for the Gateway Silver Award. She visited the home one day each week and it was decided her valuable work with the residents, mostly with Alzheimer's or dementia, should continue for the gold award. She devised a number of new ideas to stimulate and amuse them, but the most difficult and ambitious was to make a film of her friends talking about their happiest and most memorable times.

Funds were limited; so Sally used her skill as a photographer to take portraits of everyone and then tape recorded their stories. She won their full cooperation and enthusiasm from the start.

The project took many months, which tended to heighten the excitement and anticipation of everyone – but it also created concern that Sally was trying to do too much. At times during her work at the Evergreen Sally had several of her "little do's" and Sheila had to give her oxygen, which usually brought her round within 15 minutes. However, on three occasions, when Sheila was not present, an ambulance had to be called to take Sally to Scarborough Hospital for treatment before being allowed home.

Tim Stainforth, the postmaster at Thornton-le-Dale and a keen amateur cameraman, heard about Sally's film project and offered to help. Within a week he managed to transfer the Evergreen faces and voices onto videotape with soft background music chosen by Sally.

They worked together to edit it down to 45 minutes with professional-style opening and titles; and then arranged a date for the premiere on the large screen television set in the Evergreen lounge.

It would be difficult to describe the sheer delight of the

16 stars and also Evergreen owner Maureen Middleton and her staff. They all insisted that a beaming Sally take a bow at the end – before a second screening by special request of everyone.

The success of the film stimulated Sally to go on to complete all the many challenges well within the time allowed.

Soon after a letter arrived from the Gateway headquarters, congratulating Sally as the first person to achieve the Gold Award. It was to be presented to her at the joint Mencap and Gateway Conference in Blackpool on 12th November 1994.

The news was celebrated over afternoon tea and cakes at the nursing home where Gran, in a rare moment of awareness, smiled and laughed and hugged Sally. "I am so happy for you," she said.

Sadly, later that October, just a month before Sally's big day, Gran passed away peacefully.

16

Singing in the rain

The windscreen wipers on Sheila's car were going at double speed in a torrential downpour as they drove to Blackpool for Sally's golden day. It started raining as they left Thornton-le-Dale on the morning of Friday 11th November 1994, and the grey unfriendly clouds dominated and almost drowned the whole weekend.

Sally had not been in good health all week. There was even a serious doubt about her being well enough to travel, but she couldn't let anyone down, especially after the Gateway organisers had booked Becky, her faithful pet and constant companion, into the hotel by special request.

In a phone conversation the outspoken Sally told the organisers: "Becky is blind, deaf and very old. I can't come without her." The Norbreck Castle, scene of the venue, had a strict "no animals" rule; so one had to be found that welcomed pets.

In fact everything a geriatric Cavalier King Charles Spaniel required for a special seaside weekend had been carefully packed away by Sally days before the journey.

Sally was on an entertaining high all the way, reciting monologues she had learned by heart over the years to keep Sheila amused. The favourite in her repertoire, and always an instant hit, was most appropriate for her first visit to Blackpool. It was the hilarious tale of Albert and the Lion. You know … it goes something like this, and is guaranteed to help make long journeys from North Yorkshire to Lancashire seem shorter.

There's a famous seaside place called Blackpool
that's noted for fresh air and fun,
and Mr and Mrs Ramsbottom went there with
young Albert, their son.
A grand little lad was young Albert,
all dressed in his best, quite a swell
and with a stick with an 'orse's 'ead 'andle,
the finest that Woolworths could sell.
They didn't think much to the ocean,
the waves were fiddling and small,
there was no wrecks and nobody drownded,
in fact nuthing to laugh at at all.

Gateway organiser Millie Lewis and her field officer "Dolly" Gray fuelled Sally's anticipation of a very special weekend with their lavish praise for the high standard of her achievements, especially her filmed report on her work for the elderly.

Millie Lewis, who set the standards for the Duke of Edinburgh's awards before creating the Gateway challenges, believed Sally's efforts, against all odds, would become the benchmark for the scheme and an inspiration to everyone – including her Gateway team.

Sally decided at the outset it would be wrong to include her painting in her bid for gold. "It wouldn't be fair to win an award for something I already do well," she insisted.

So none of the watercolours which had brought her instant fame were on show in Blackpool. Sally had her own special stand devoted to presentations of her work over the two years of the Gateway Gold challenge. It was also arranged for her to meet Lord Rix, President of Mencap, at her stand to explain everything on show.

Sally's was just one of the many stands on display at the Norbreck Hotel where about 1,000 people from all over the UK had assembled for the first joint Gateway and Mencap Conference that wet weekend. The highlight of the Saturday evening carnival-style dinner-dance and cabaret was to be the presentation of the gold award to Sally. The timing of it and the manner was to be the surprise.

However, the first surprise for Sally on arrival in

Blackpool was to discover "Dolly" Gray, who had written several letters to her, was not a lady but a tall, muscular former Royal Marine. He explained any doubt about his gender was because of a tradition in the Marines. Anyone unlucky enough to be called Gray swiftly acquires the nickname from the popular Boer War song, "Goodbye Dolly Gray".

No one in the vast dining room at the Norbreck Hotel had any idea Sally had collapsed earlier while walking on the sea front and had to be revived with oxygen. After sleeping all afternoon she felt well enough for the party, but was still unaware her presentation was to be the highlight of the evening.

Sally could never be a fashion icon, clamped in callipers and with her bright red surgical boots, but she felt confident in a long black velour skirt, white silk blouse and narrow red headband to match her footwear.

Throughout her life all Sally's food had to be liquidised; so special arrangements had been made for her to enjoy her dinner at a table set in the centre of the ballroom. In her diary she recalled the balloons floating from every chair, special lighting effects including the vast stage lit with sparkling silver stars. "The cabaret was great and there was such a warm and friendly feeling. It was a lovely evening, the best in my life. Magical," she wrote, "I felt all the hard work was so worthwhile."

After dinner and the last cabaret act the lights dimmed and there was a roll of drums, "Suddenly there was a spotlight on our table, settling on me," she recalled. "I felt a hand on my shoulder and I looked up and it was Lord Rix who told everyone, 'this is our special guest, Sally Johnson, a remarkable young lady who is our first Gateway Gold award winner.' Everyone started clapping and a voice called for three cheers for me. I felt like I'd just scored a winning goal for Manchester United in the Cup Final."

Sally responded in her usual way, raising more cheers when she threw her arms into the air and shouted, "Wheyhey. I've done it!"

She wrote: "It was a natural reaction. I'd watched sporting stars do it on television. It seemed the best way to thank everyone for being so kind. I had a first dance with Dolly Gray and then so many others; and in between folk came up to congratulate me. I felt I was dreaming it all. It was lovely."

The party continued until 2.00 a.m. but soon after midnight Sally was fast asleep in bed at their hotel after relating all her happy memories to dear old Becky.

Her final diary note on the weekend: "We sang all the way back home. It was still raining heavily. It never stopped, but there was nothing but sunshine in our hearts."

17

Make each day special

As all the medical opinion on Sally's immediate future became increasingly negative Sheila decided the only positive response was to travel.

There were so many places they hadn't seen, or others to visit again, even on the nearby North Yorkshire Moors and in the Dales they loved so much. They had never explored the mysteries of Snowdonia in North Wales, which became their first destination. Sally had fond memories of an earlier visit to South Wales and a new tourist attraction there. It was a disued coalmine and, after going down in the cage, a hefty guide, an ex-miner, carried her on his shoulders and called her "Sugar Sal".

Cumbria and the Lakes, Northumbria and Scotland, Sally's favourite, beckoned also as they spent hours over maps and guide books that late spring.

What was the alternative? Staying at home, living a claustrophobic existence in Ebor Cottage and pushing Sally around the village in her wheelchair only on sunny days? It was too gloomy to even consider. Sheila decided their lives must now be lived to the full, not soured in empty or despairing thoughts.

Sally's physical body was on borrowed time, but her mind was still bright, alert and inquiring. The love and stimulation her family had given from the day she was born was as vital now to her well-being as food and drink and the oxygen that kept her alive.

It was time to think about having a long holiday together

without a care in the world, all carefully planned but, as always, open to instant re-think.

Becoming a couch potato, desperately flicking around the TV channels all day was a non-starter. They had the will to get up and go. They had a need to create their own drama and excitement – even with the portable oxygen cylinder always at hand for Sally's "little do's".

Somehow, no matter the weather, days always seemed sunny for Sheila and Sally when they were out and about in the countryside, exploring what most folk tend to take for granted. Like all artists they needed to examine the light and shade of simple but ever-present values in life. The drama, mysteries, excitement, tranquillity and joy Mother Nature offers so freely to those who seek them, or are prepared to open their eyes and minds to her wonders.

Sheila knew the fresh clean air – and everything else on offer – would help Sally cope with her pain and stay alive and with her a little longer. Each day would be a bonus. Besides, the relentless pressures of being Sally's loving mum, best friend and carer, would be eased. The repeated dashes for oxygen and long nights of fitful sleep were beginning to take their toll on Sheila's health. But the never-ending drive to put purpose and fun into Sally's life also stimulated her own senses, helping to make the heartache more bearable.

The long summer break was kind to all their hopes and dreams – and also Sally's fragile health. She started painting again on their first jaunt to the Dales, basing themselves in Dent Dale, source of so many friends, happy days – and inspiration.

One day, as they were busy sketching an old stone barn, Sally put down her pencil and suddenly started to create a picture in words that Sheila hastily scribbled down on the back of her pad. Sally called it 'The Old Barn'.

> The old barn stands in sad decay
> Beside the hedge all strewn with May
> The swallows build between the eaves

A sycamore strews it with her leaves
The owl has brought her young to flight
The mice the owl has put to fright
And in among the crooked beams
I see a spider's web still gleams
And through the cracked and broken beams
A golden shaft of sunlight gleams
And dappled on the dusty floor
Spreads outwards from the broken door.

Sally loved Shakespeare, Burns, Wordsworth and Tennyson and at times she would suddenly create and recite her own verse. "Somehow she always seemed to burst into verse when I was driving and unable to get it down in writing," says Sheila. "Some were quite inspiring, but Sally could never remember them later to record them. She claimed the flow of words 'just came into my head. I don't know how or where they came from', she'd say."

One of their many day trips was to the Stump Cross Caverns, near Pately Bridge, but they got a cold reception at the ticket office when Sheila asked for two admissions. The lady behind the counter was typical West Yorkshire, blunt but friendly with it. She stared at Sally's obvious disability and pulled a wry face, shaking her head at the same time.

"How do you think you're going to get that young lass down there?" she demanded.

"I'll carry her piggy back," said Sheila.

"You won't you know. Not down 87 steps … and that's the easiest bit … and you've got to climb up 'em again," she said. "You'll never do it. Not carrying your daughter on your back. Don't try … even think about it. If I sell you tickets it'll be my responsibility if summat happens to you."

But Sheila had already hoisted Sally onto her back and was on her way, saying, "Don't worry. I'll take the risk and any responsibility – and I'll pay you when we get back."

They saw all the spectacular stalactites and stalagmites, the full tour, and after carrying Sally up those 87 steps Sheila was hot and tired. She paused to get her breath before saying, "Two tickets, please."

The woman laughed and came out from behind the counter to give Sheila a big hug. "It's on the house, luv. You've earned it," she said and gave Sally a free guidebook.

There was a sadness for Sally and Sheila during those happy days. Becky, Sally's pet Cavalier spaniel, passed away peacefully in her 15th year. But soon after Auntie Pat bought her a new male Cavalier, called Darcy. He arrived towards the end of the brilliant BBC television adaptation of *Pride and Prejudice* starring Colin Firth as the handsome, intensely romantic Mr Darcy. Sally's new companion was also handsome, and to her great delight her Darcy turned out to be a loveable delinquent, but entertaining with it, and totally devoted to her.

Ferry-hopping from the Scottish mainland around the rugged Western Isles was enchanting and tiring for Sheila and Sally but they decided they had, at last, found their idyllic holiday location, a rented cottage at the water's edge on the Isle of Arran.

The joy of discovery almost turned to tragedy within hours of arriving when Sally collapsed and Sheila dashed for the oxygen cylinder in the car. As Sally's face turned an alarming blue and she fought for each breath Sheila held the oxygen mask to her face. "It'll soon be all right, Sally," she whispered as she was about to open the valve.

To her horror she realised it was already open and the cylinder was empty. It had been used by Sheila a few times during the holiday and also by Sally when she felt she needed a boost. Somehow, obviously by accident, the valve had been left open.

Sheila quickly realised she had no choice but to leave Sally and find a phone box to call for help. Thankfully, after running for only a few minutes, which seemed like hours, she found a cottage with a phone.

It was a Sunday with only one doctor on duty. He was on call at the other side of the island, but responded as quickly as he could to pick up a replacement cylinder and drive to the cottage.

For an agonising twenty minutes Sheila held Sally in her arms, praying as she watched her gasp for air and waiting for the young GP who could save her.

Within seconds of his arrival the life-saving oxygen was flowing and the blue pallor began to leave Sally's cheeks as her breathing became more relaxed.

Some years earlier her local GP gave Sheila a sealed letter to carry with her wherever they went, detailing Sally's medical history and medication. "It would be helpful for another doctor in an emergency," he said. It had never been opened until that day on Arran. It told the Scottish doctor about her many problems and went on: "Here is a life worth saving. In her short life Sally has achieved more than most of us achieve in a lifetime."

Their holiday continued to fulfil all their expectations and more, especially the many kindnesses of the friendly islanders. "Theirs is such a hard and simple life," Sally wrote in her diary, "But they are enriched with what really matters in life."

Some time later they decided to return to Arran to thank everyone who had been so kind and helpful to them.

The year proved a tonic for both with so many happy memories of treasured experiences, people and places. It was to help them through some dark, troubled months ahead when Sheila suddenly became ill.

She always joked she could never find time to be ill, but she had a harsh warning when she fell asleep at the wheel of her car. It was on a short journey to Bridlington with Sally to spend the day with Pat. Sheila just nodded off, but somehow managed to brake hard as the car skidded off the road. She and Sally escaped with only a sharp shock.

It had almost happened before but Sheila never mentioned it to anyone. She decided she was perhaps a little run-down, but now she felt scared it could be something worse when she began to suffer frequent migraines and blurred vision. Her GP urged her to take a break, a total rest from the 24-hour care she gave Sally. He sent her to see a specialist who recommended a permanent break from her daughter as the only solution.

Within a system that rarely favours carers the £37 a week allowance Sheila had received for caring for Sally was snatched away when she received her old age pension. She needed help with the housework to attend to Sally's many needs, but couldn't afford it and was advised to contact Social Services. "It would be one thing less to worry about," she said. The unacceptable response was: "We can only arrange for someone to look after Sally while you do your housework."

The only immediate but short-term solution was for Sally to go twice a week to the Cauwood Day Centre in Malton which gave Sheila time to catch up with a backlog of chores, leaving her even more exhausted.

Now she lay awake at night worried not only about Sally but also about her own health and future. What if she found she couldn't cope any longer? What if she died? Who would look after Sally? Where could she find around-the-clock nursing care, which she now needed, except in a nursing home for the old and frail? Her questions brought on disturbing nightmares when she did manage to sleep.

It couldn't end like that, she decided, after all they had been through together. She wouldn't let it happen and in her deeply unhappy state she prayed desperately for the unthinkable.

"Please, God, let Sally die before me."

Her prayers were answered in a happier way when Sally was offered respite at the Wilf Ward Trust's Isabella Court in nearby Pickering, just a day or two at a time.

But as Sheila's health improved slowly, Sally's worsened rapidly.

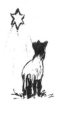

18

A bright light

Sally loved the BBC's early Sunday evening programme *Songs of Praise*, and was delighted when it included her favourite hymns.

She would sing along with them and joke to Sheila: "I'll have that one at my funeral. Lovely tune. Everyone can sing that."

The family had been engulfed with sadness with the passing of Ken, Gran, and, of course, the problems of severely handicapped Auntie Pat, living alone in Bridlington.

Sheila and Sally believed death was not the end but a journey to a better place. They also felt that while they lived their thoughts should always be with the living; and as Christians, they should always be willing to help those in need.

The only secret kept from Sally was that her condition was terminal. It demanded a reassuring calm from Sheila every time Sally collapsed at home, in the supermarket, or in the countryside. She relied on the oxygen to pull Sally back from the brink. It went everywhere with them.

It takes a special kind of courage to watch an only child appear to die, often several times a day. One day, as she recovered from a collapse, Sally started talking about seeing Jesus in what appeared to be a religious experience. Sheila recalls: "As she regained consciousness her face was glowing with happiness."

In a hushed voice Sally told her: "I was walking down a dark tunnel when suddenly there was a bright light. As I walked towards it I heard a voice saying 'Come to me Sally, come to me.' I saw Jesus and I ran into his arms. I was able to run for the first time in my life. Jesus said: 'There's no need to be afraid. I'll look after you'."

Sally recorded everything about her experience the same day in the diary she kept to help her write her book one day.

She had been so close to death before. If what she recounted was an over-fertile imagination why had it never happened before? The religious experience comforted Sheila as they prepared for another Christmas together. But she also sensed Sally was now aware she was living on borrowed time.

Somehow Sally always saw Christmas through the eyes of a child, without accepting or seeking the commercial gloss. She even pretended to believe there was a Father Christmas and never seemed to lose that sense of childish awe and excitement over the birth of Jesus.

The folk in Thornton-le-Dale loved Sally for her generous and lively spirit which seemed to be with her all year round. They also worried about her well-being and in 1992, after one of her life-threatening health scares, they gave her the honour of switching on the village Christmas lights. They felt it could be her last Christmas and wanted it to be a very special evening.

Their love and kind thoughts for her were, of course, seven years premature, but they weren't aware of this at the time.

Sally arrived on the sleigh with Santa, waving to the crowds before flicking the switch. And, as the thousands of coloured light bulbs blazed to brighten the frosty air, there was a resounding cheer for Sally – and tears from those who feared the worst for her.

Now in 1999 her thoughts were on the Millennium as she joined the crowds around the village cross in her wheelchair, full of enthusiasm but weak and very tired. It was to be Sally's last Christmas among all her friends in the village she loved.

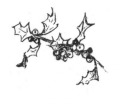

19

Dark shadow

'A Prickly Landing' for the DSA's Christmas 2000 card was Sally's last painting, completed despite failing eyesight and the searing pain of gout in her hands and wrists.

Her energy levels had also dropped alarmingly and she could barely walk the length of the garden path from the back door of Ebor Cottage to the garage.

But her sense of humour remained. "I'm sure this path is getting longer," she would joke as she shuffled along, stopping several times to gasp for breath. At times she couldn't walk at all because of her pain. Sheila had to lift her on and off the stairlift and often carry her wherever they went.

Sally's blackouts were also becoming more frequent and doctors discovered her blood had thickened to a critical level. The only treatment for this was to take a pint away every few weeks to try to thin it down.

Early in 2000 the members of the Down's Syndrome Association presented Sally with a special achievement award. Everyone was also delighted with the sense of fun in her painting of the cheeky robin about to land on a prickly holly leaf.

Sally was thrilled to hear, on 17th April, that it was with the printers with an order for 40,000 copies of the year 2000 Christmas card. It went on sale to become a huge success with demand finally outstripping supply and making a profit of £12,000 for DSA funds.

The news was the perfect reason for a modest celebration, a trip by car the next day to Sally's favourite tearoom in Wykeham. She loved their special coffee and besides, she and Sheila felt Darcy, Sally's devoted pet, would enjoy an afternoon scampering about in a nearby forest. The sun shone for them on one of their happiest days.

Good news can be a tonic and the glowing letter from the DSA had given Sally's health a big lift. There was no need to use the oxygen cylinder all afternoon and a beaming Sally said: "I feel so well, Sheila, better than I have for months."

Over coffee they talked about everything and everyone, but mostly their impending trip to Scotland which Sheila had booked knowing Sally might be too ill to travel. She felt they both needed something positive to look forward to, and now it was only four weeks away.

Sally had learned to love Scotland and the Scots, was fascinated by its history and more especially in the life and times, poems and songs, of Rabbie Burns. After visiting his home and museum in Ayrshire she felt inspired to paint pictures in words when her hands were unable to use brushes for any length of time. One of her best pieces of blank verse was 'Autumn'. Sally never wasted time trying to work out a long title and her blank verse often reads like a visual for a new painting.

> Trees on fire with Autumn glow,
> brilliant sunlight touching the branches,
> bird calls rippling through the air,
> country smells amidst the crackling leaves,
> which quiver in the breeze,
> creating a tremor in the peace and tranquillity,
> bright red hips studding and livening the bankside,
> adding colour to the lushness of the grasses,
> this is Autumn.

Next day, 19th April, Sally became desperately ill and in so much pain the doctor visited the cottage three times. She rallied in the afternoon, enough to eat a little and watch some television, but Sheila had a deeper sense of foreboding than ever before.

She also felt a need to cuddle her, holding her tight to avoid a dark shadow about to eclipse their world.

"Oh Sally," she said, holding back her tears. "I wish I could bear the pain for you, darling." How often had she thought and said that over the years, but Sally's response was always the same – and with a smile.

"You can't, but you do help me to bear it. Come on, let's play dominoes. I fancy a game." Sally would come up with something like this to defuse any fears Sheila had about her welfare.

They played six games, winning three each before Sally, who was tiring fast, said: "Let's call it a draw. I'm ready for my bed."

She made a move towards the stairway but collapsed on the way. She appeared to recover momentarily, but fainted again and then a third time. As Sheila held her in her arms Sally whispered: "I just can't cope any more.".

Sheila tried frantically to revive her, as she had so many times before, but quickly realised it wasn't going to work. She picked up the telephone to call the doctor and ambulance, but somehow her fingers began to dial the number of Janet Magee, Methodist Minister and friend.

Before the number rang out the front door opened suddenly and Janet walked in to immediately give comfort and quietly take control.

Within minutes the ambulance and doctor arrived and Sheila felt the numbing effect of what she had always known would happen one day.

It seemed that suddenly the house was full and then, one by one, everyone departed until she was alone. The cottage, filled for so many years with the light and joy of Sally's chatter, was silent. She had somehow seemed invincible, having cheated death from the day she was born.

As news of Sally's death spread a deluge of cards arrived, hundreds of them expressing sorrow and praise for a short life that had reached out to so many and achieved so much. The sadness of her passing was felt around the world.

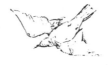

20

Back to Dent Dale

It was no surprise to Sheila to find Sally had planned her own funeral, all clearly written down in her diary on which this book is based.

The Methodist church was packed with those who knew and loved her, to recall her charm and courage – and to sing out her favourite hymns: How Great Thou Art, The Servant King and Great Is Thy Faithfulness.

Sally, always one for the big occasion, would have loved it, said Minister Janet Magee, whose portrait of Sally was a powerful example of life lived to the full but always with faith, hope and joy.

Sally's best friend, Ben Moss, who overcame his own disabilities to become a valued member of the staff at nearby Flamingo Land Theme Park and Zoo, gave an emotional reading of the 23rd Psalm, a final, moving farewell.

Afterwards villagers and friends celebrated Sally's life and memories of her at a reception in the church hall as Sheila travelled with the coffin to the Crematorium for a final farewell.

Poor Darcy, Sally's much loved pet, searched every room for her, as dogs tend to do after losing a companion, and he listened for many weeks, hoping to hear her voice.

In the Autumn Sheila took Darcy with her to Dent Dale to scatter Sally's ashes at her favourite place; and quietly recall the happy times they shared together as a family.

She was proud of all that Sally achieved in a short life which at birth seemed a tragedy only to become a triumph with her paintings selling around the world for charities; and displayed from an orphanage in Albania to a Prime Minister's study in 10 Downing Street, London.

Sally Johnson will be remembered not only as an inspirational child, but a wonderful, funny, intelligent companion and a caring, loving daughter.

Sheila's daughter. Her baby. A face like a flower.